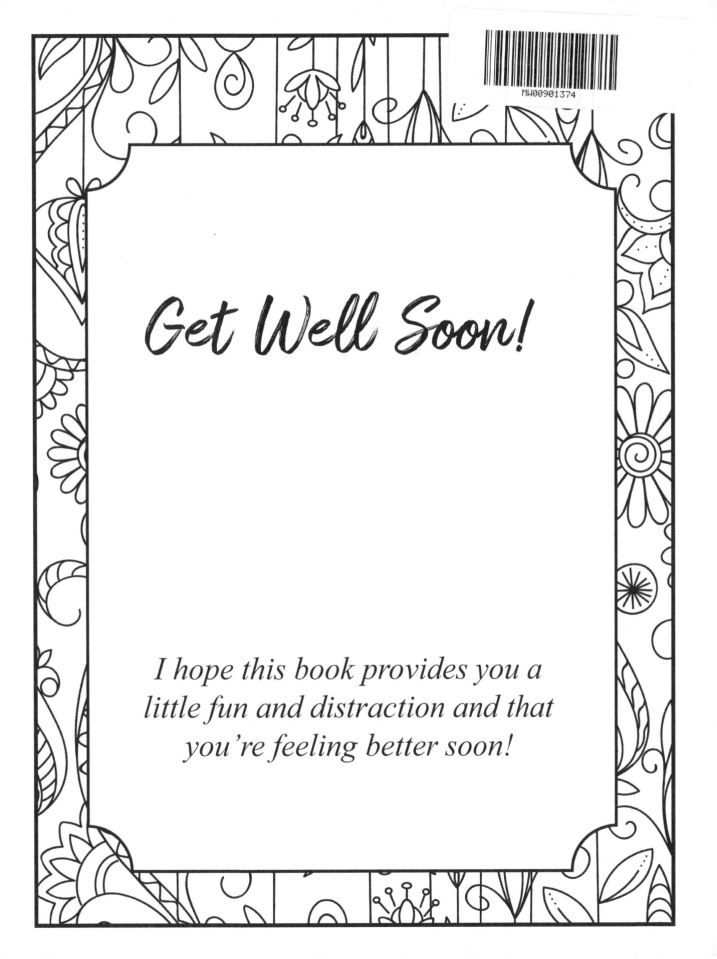

Get Well Soon!

*I hope this book provides you a
little fun and distraction and that
you're feeling better soon!*

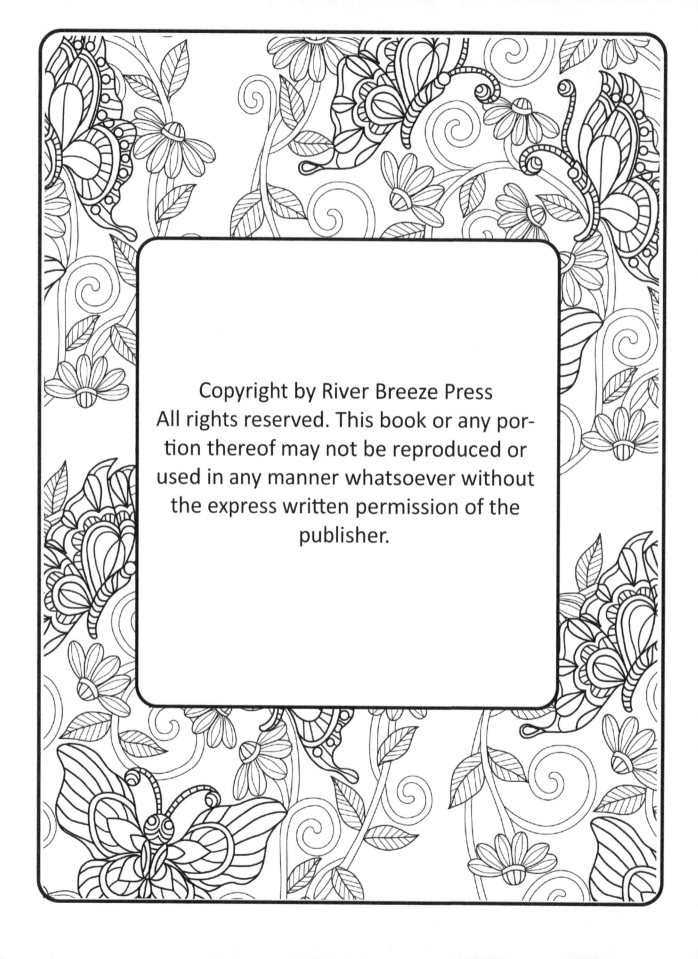

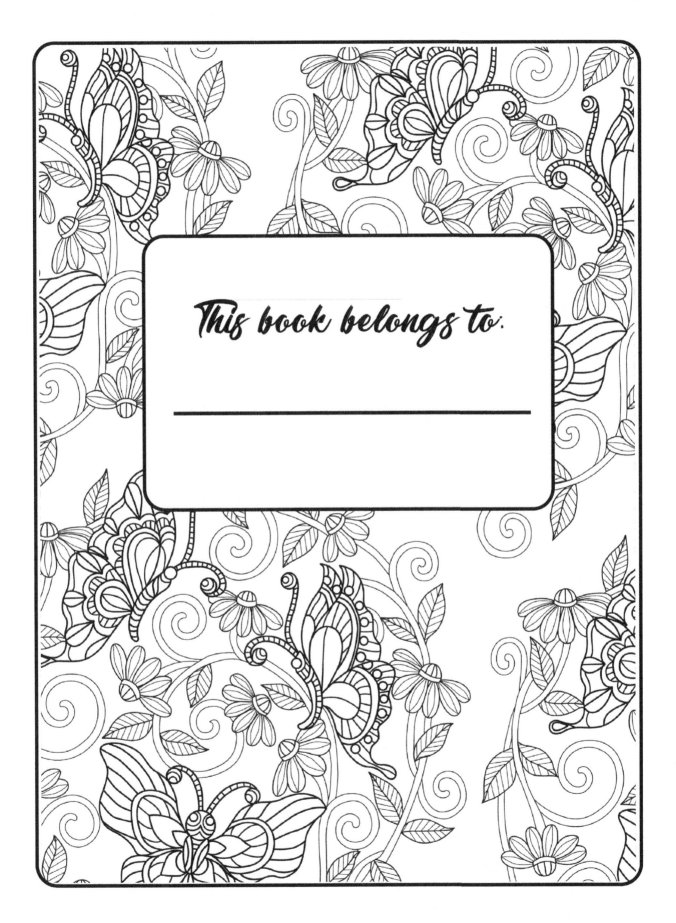

This book belongs to:

_____

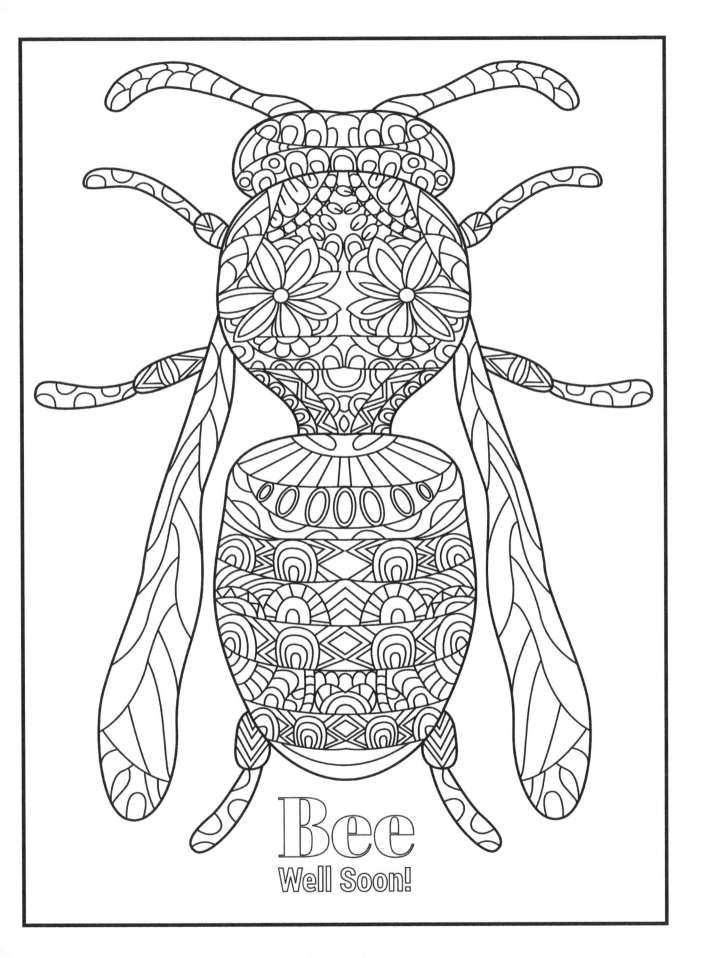

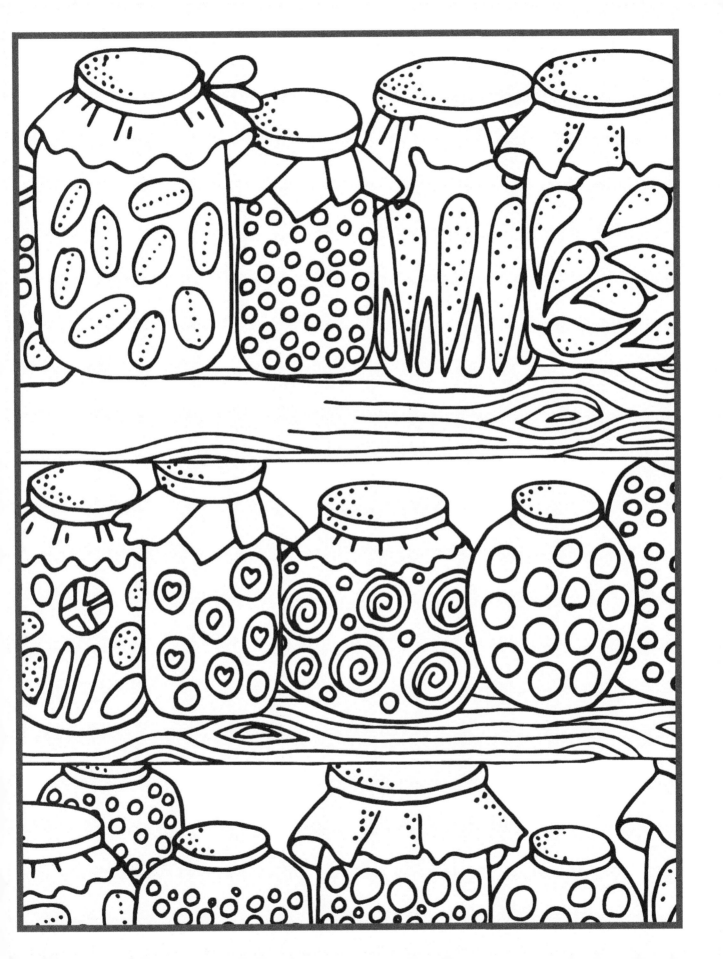

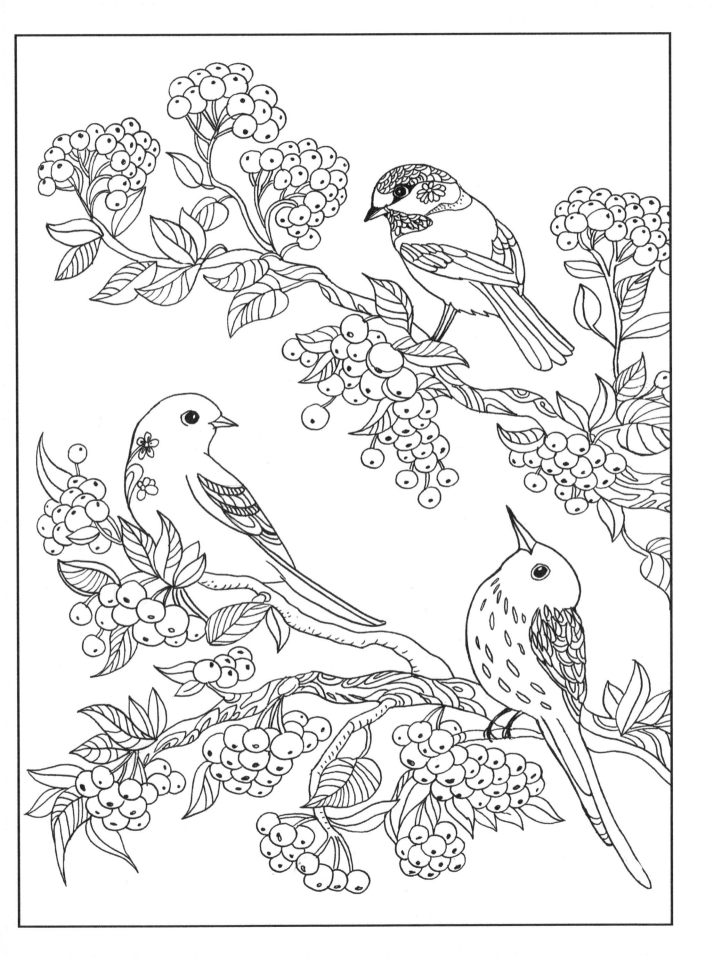

SORRY YOU FEEL WAFFLE

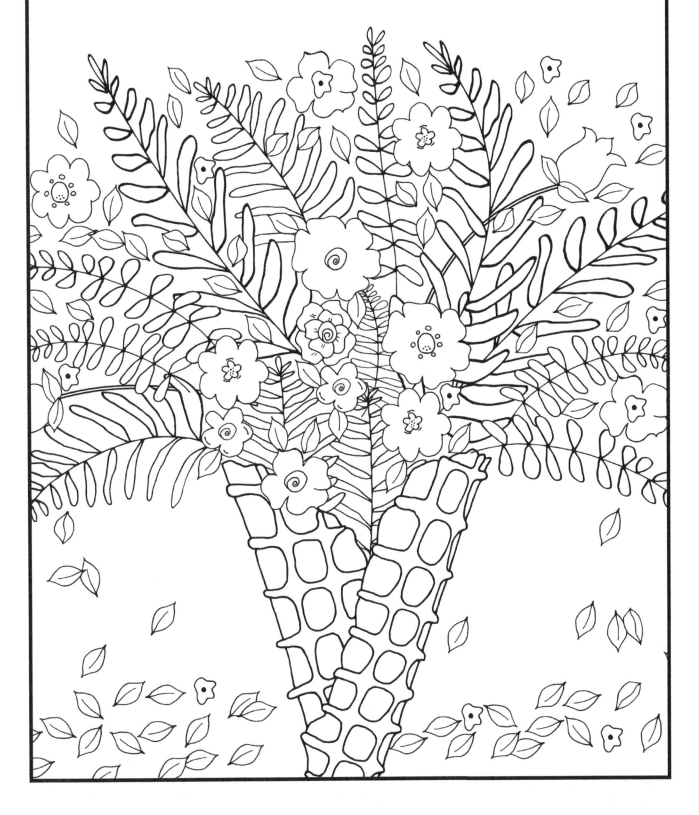

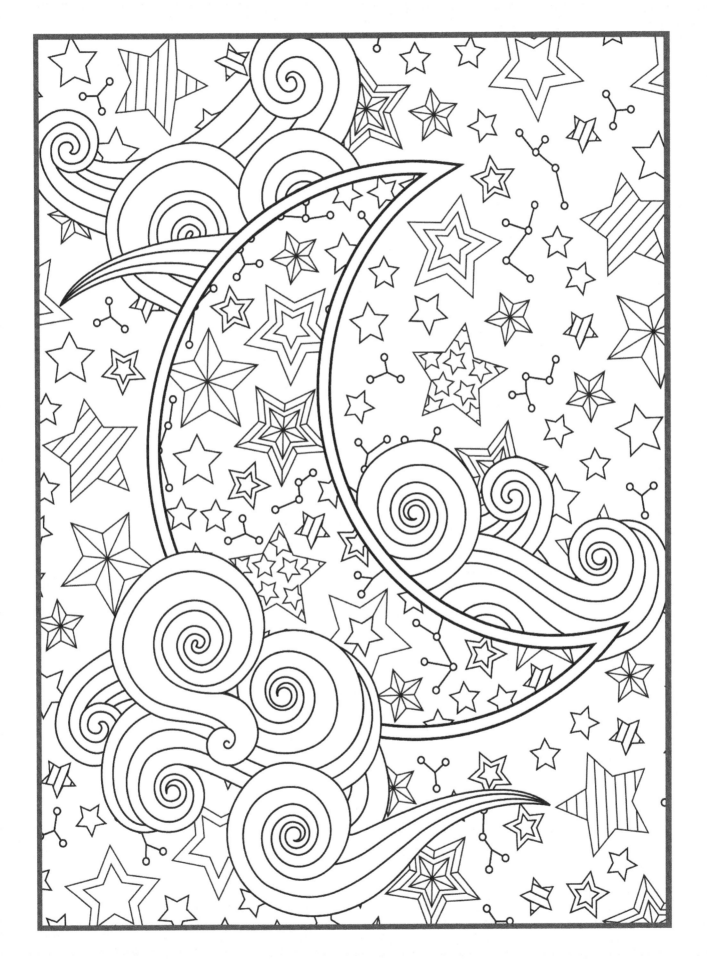

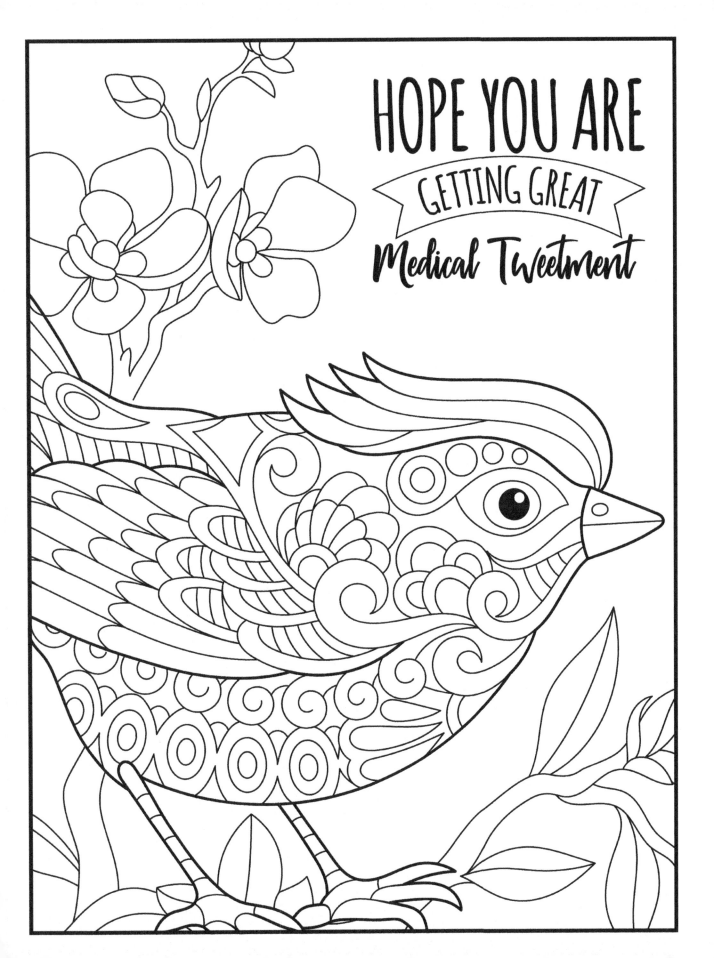

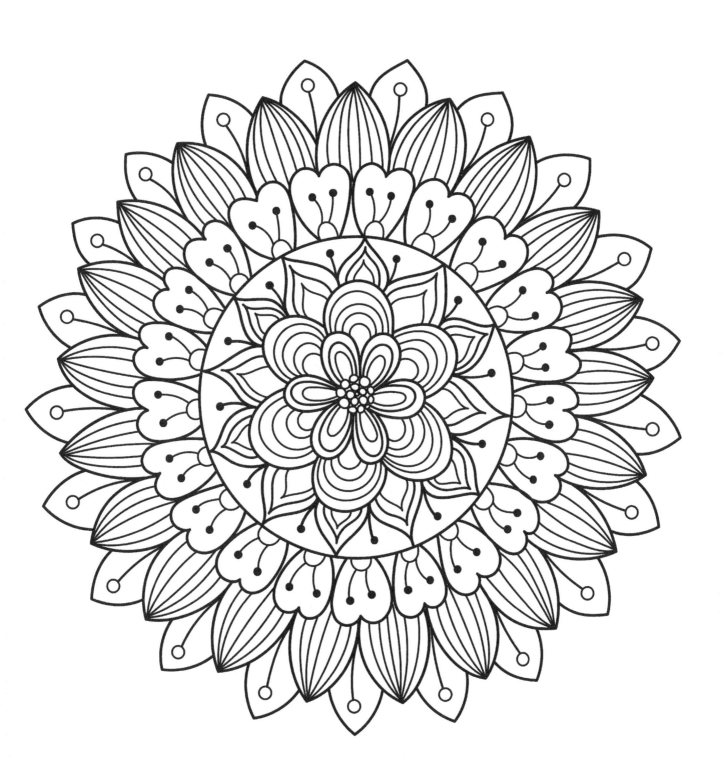

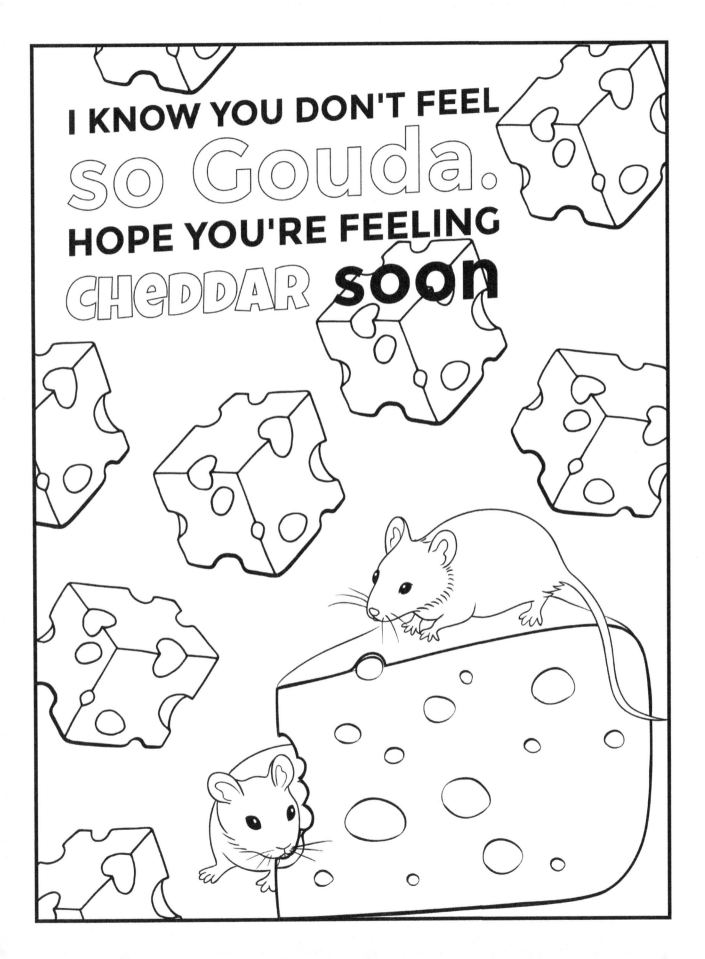

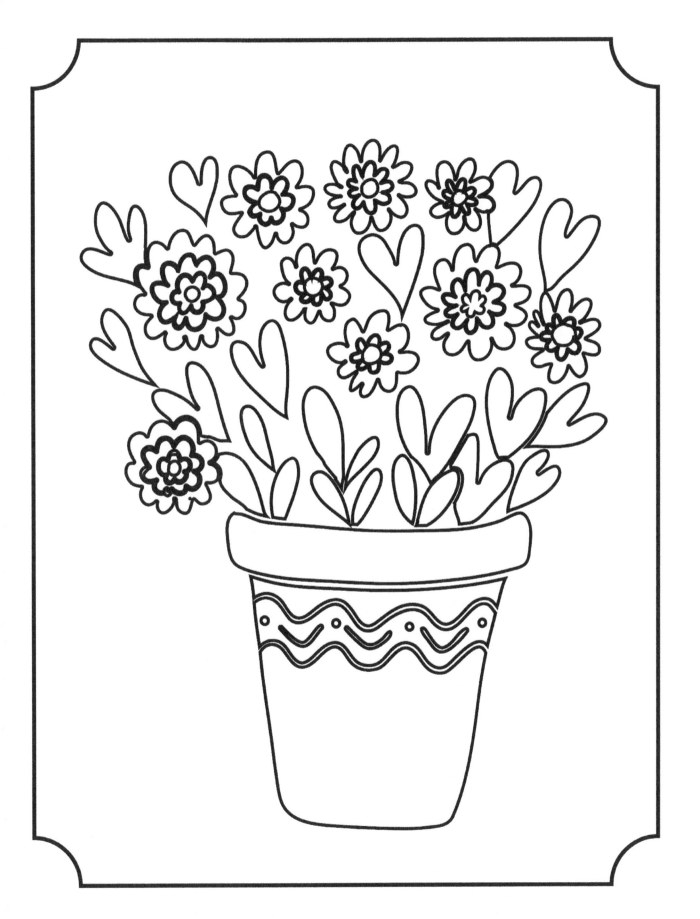

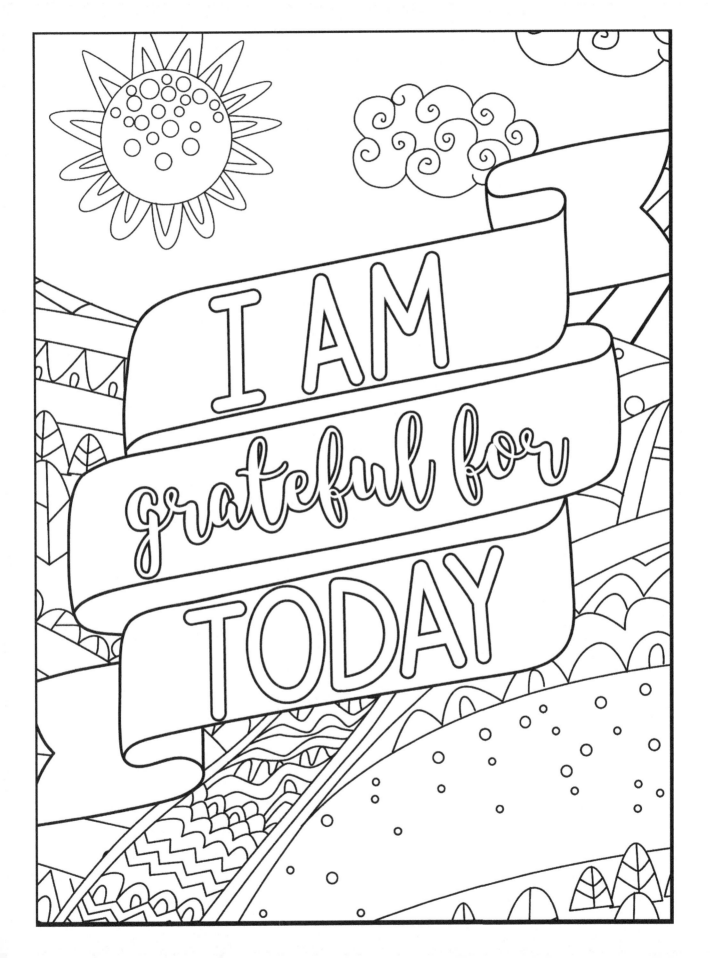

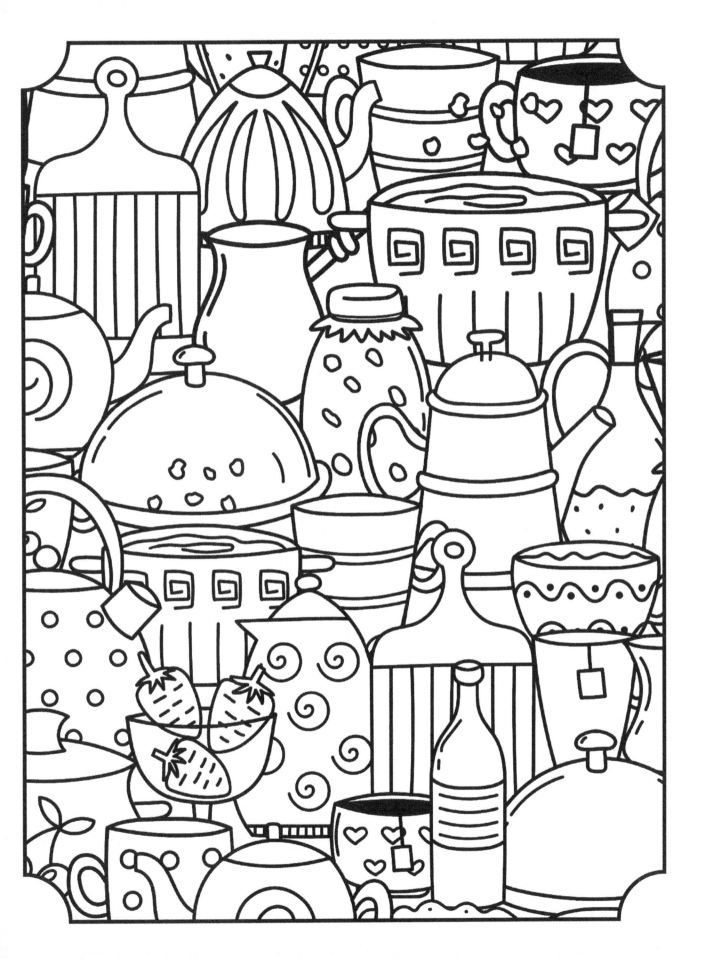

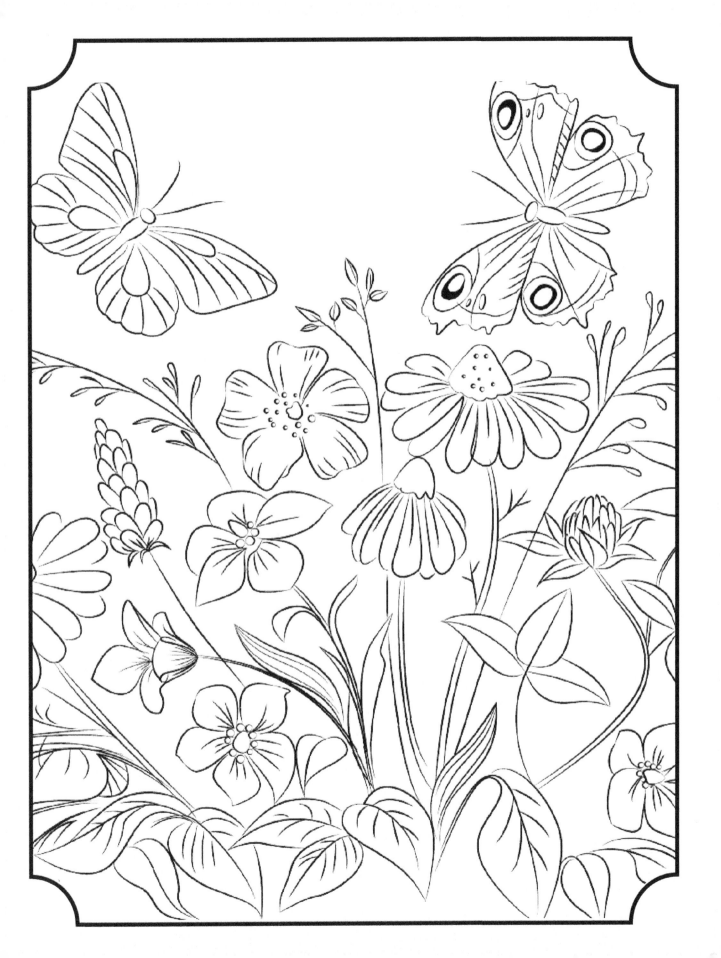

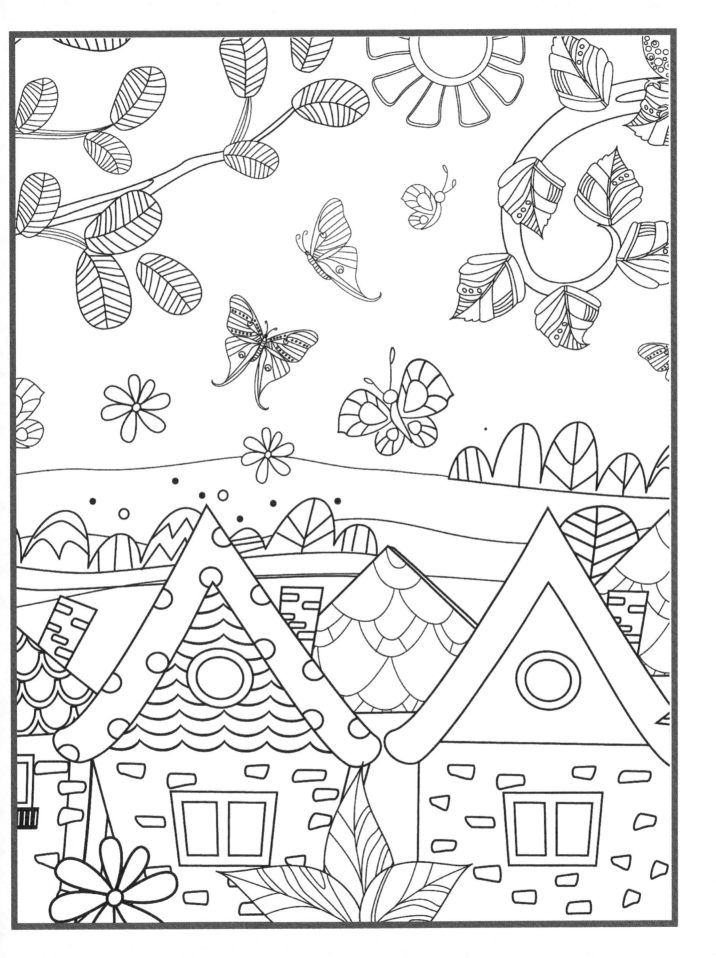

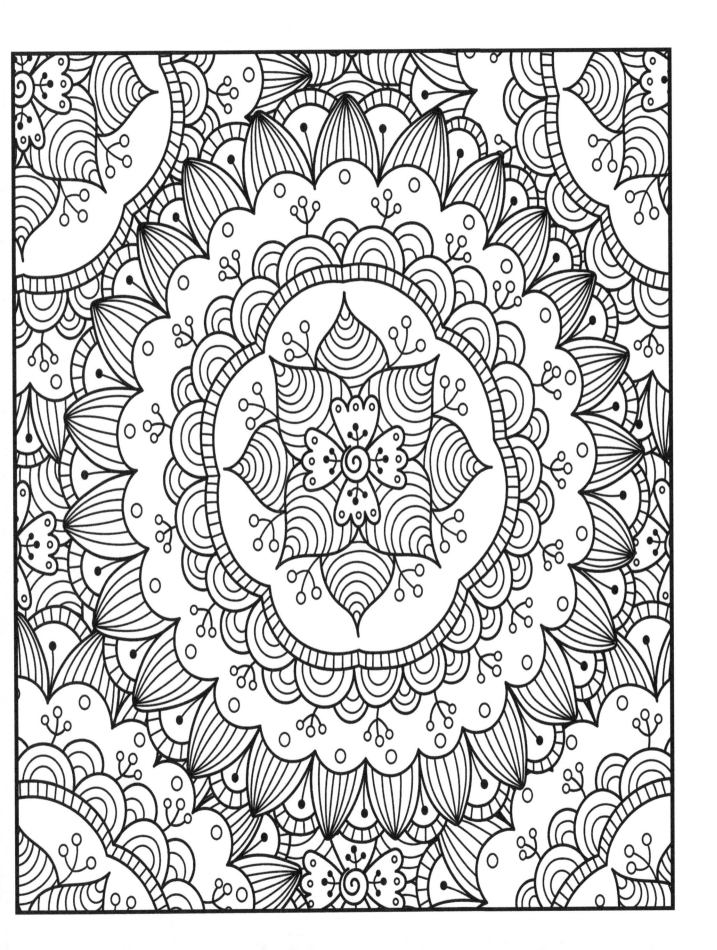

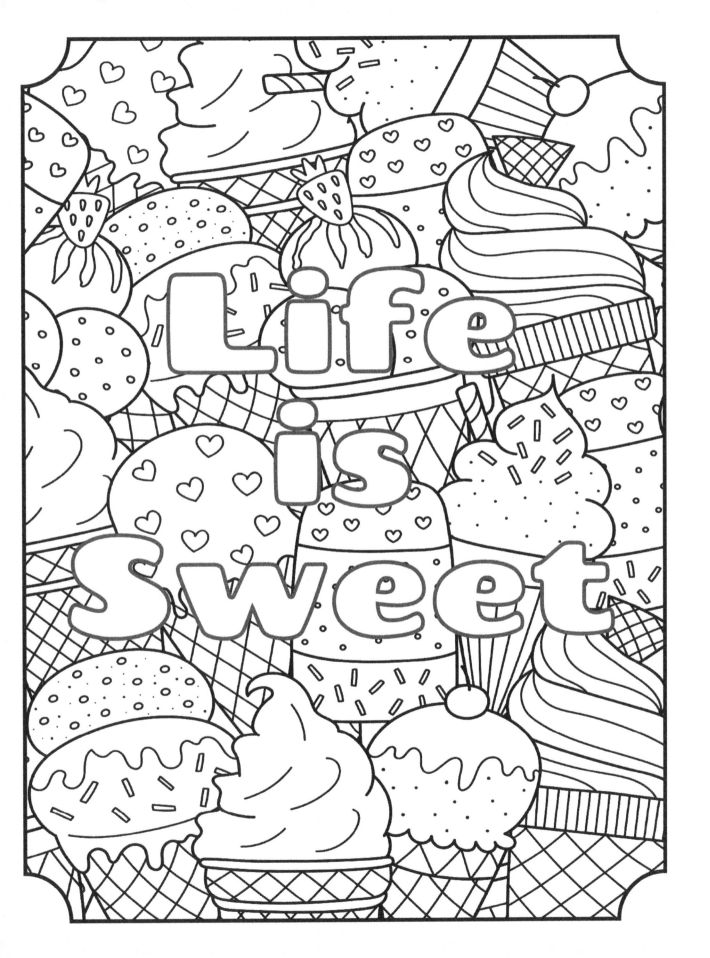

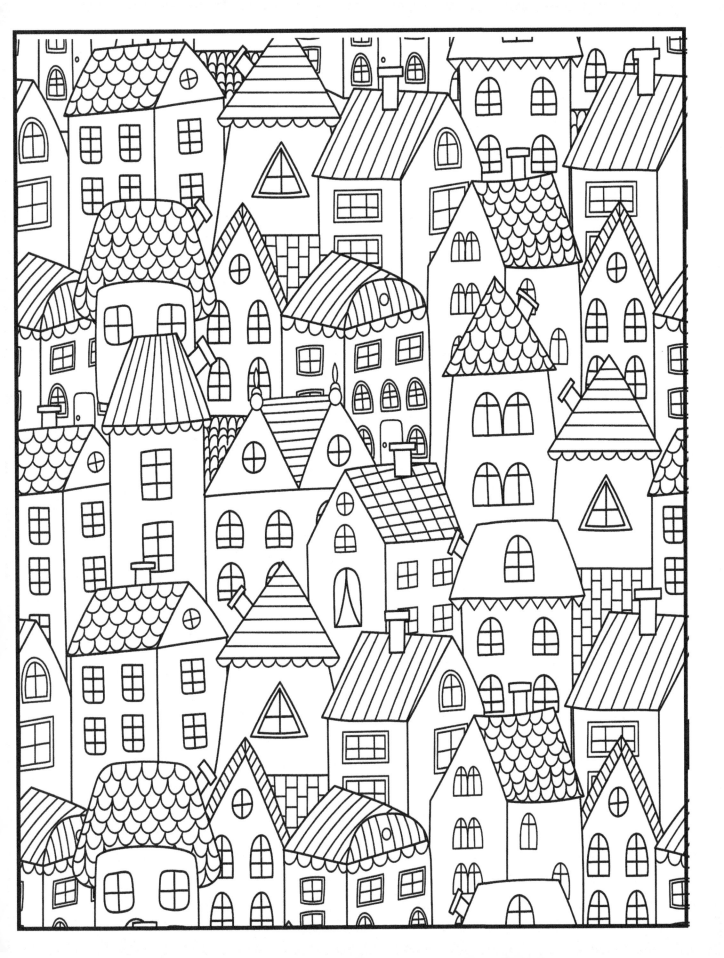

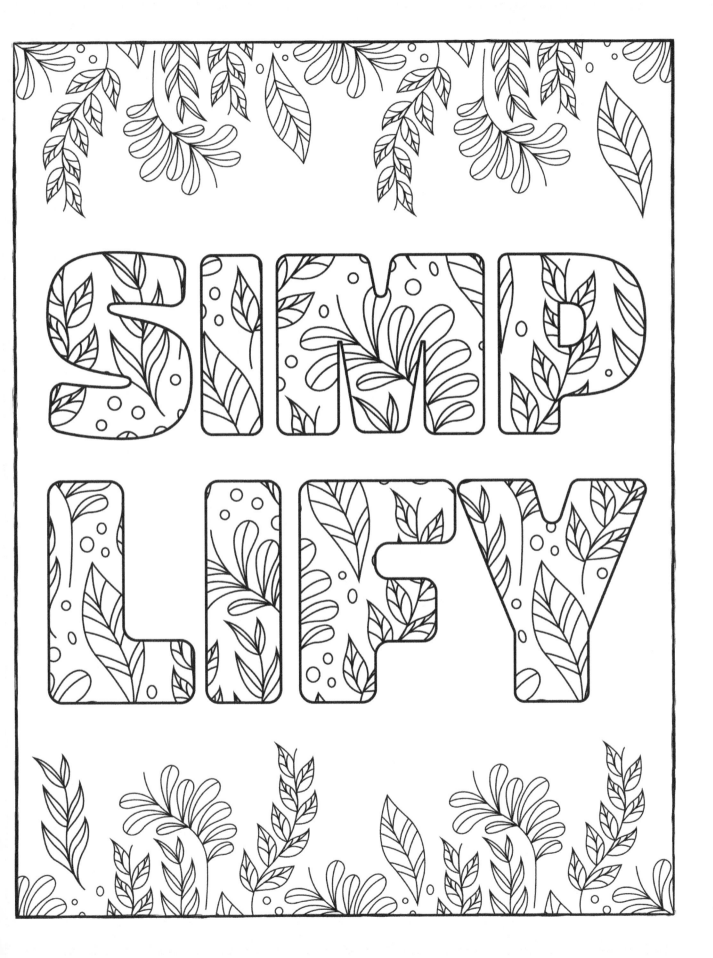

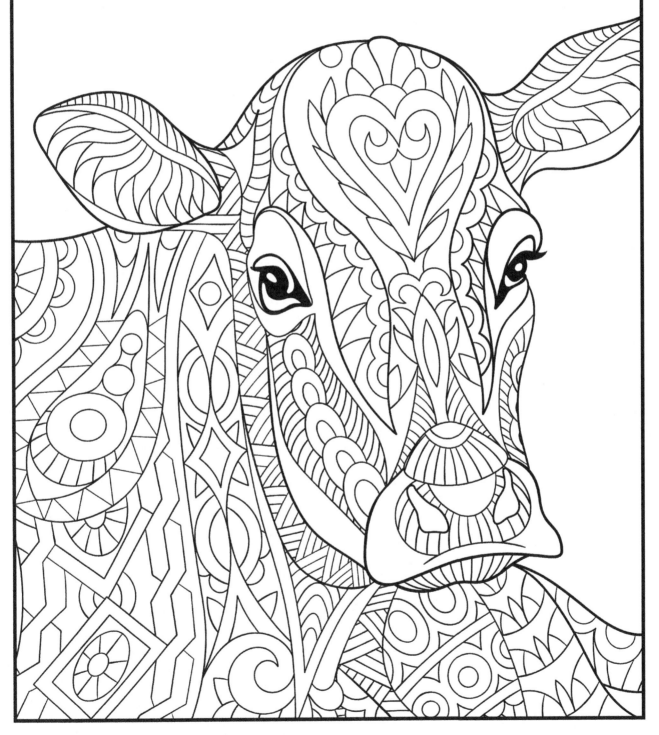

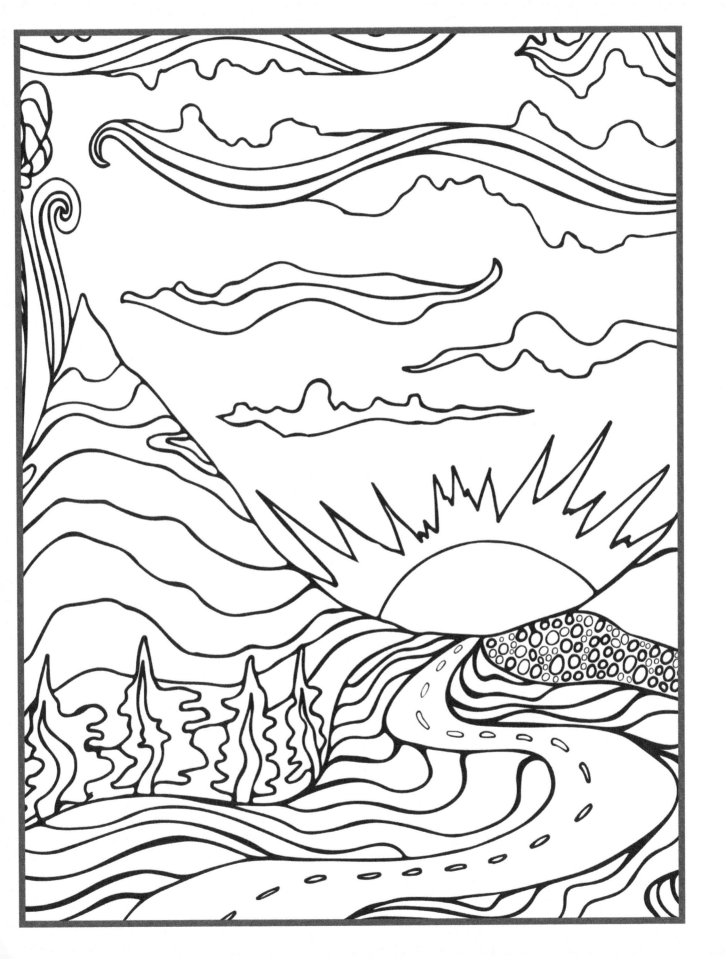

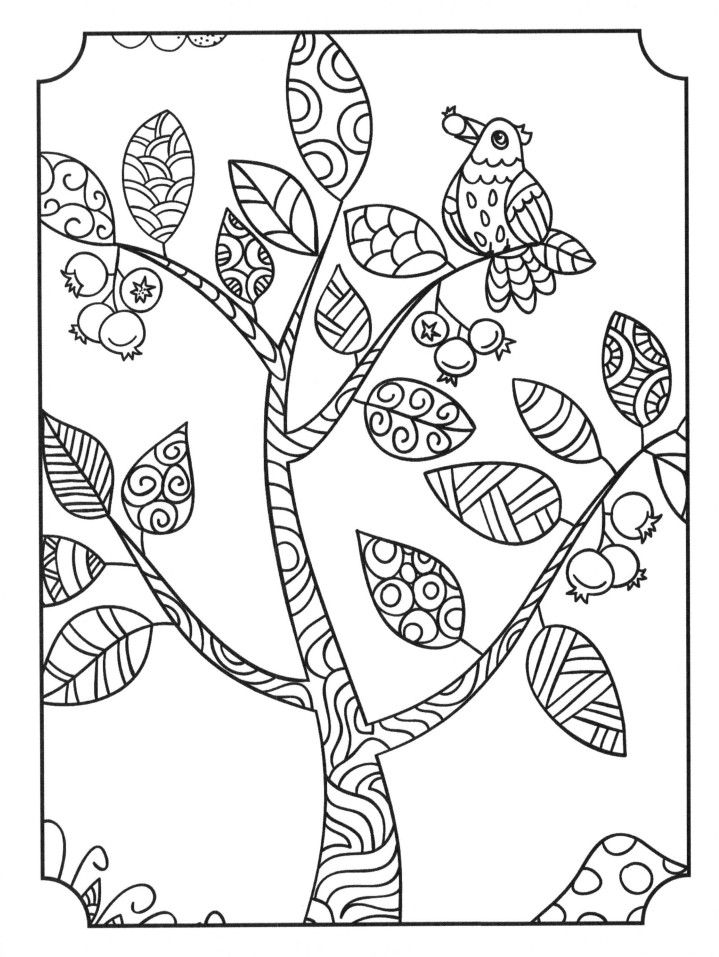

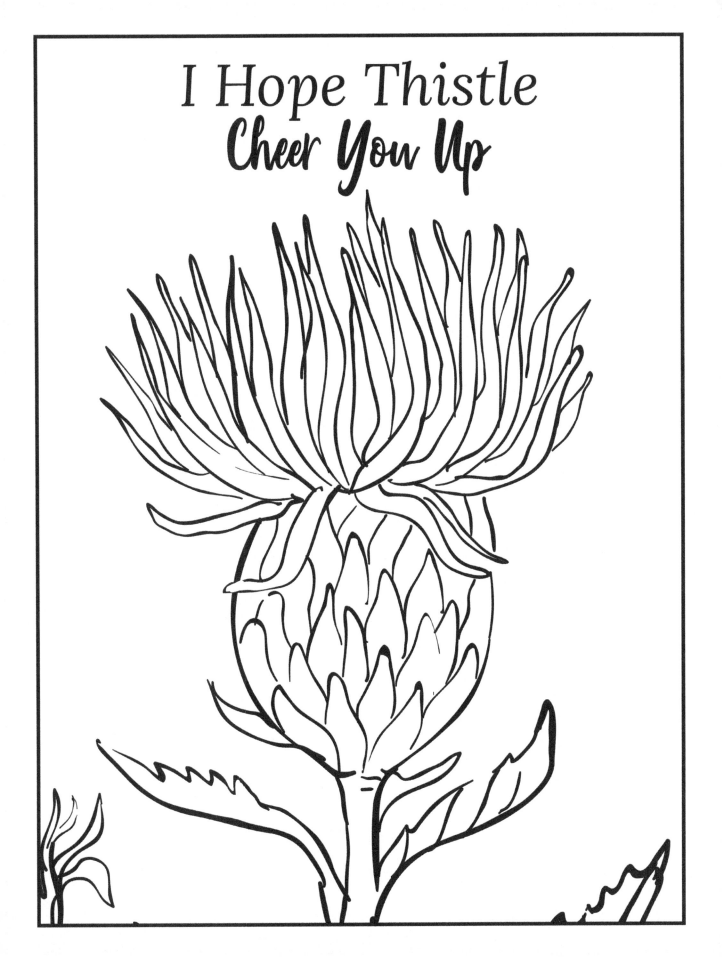

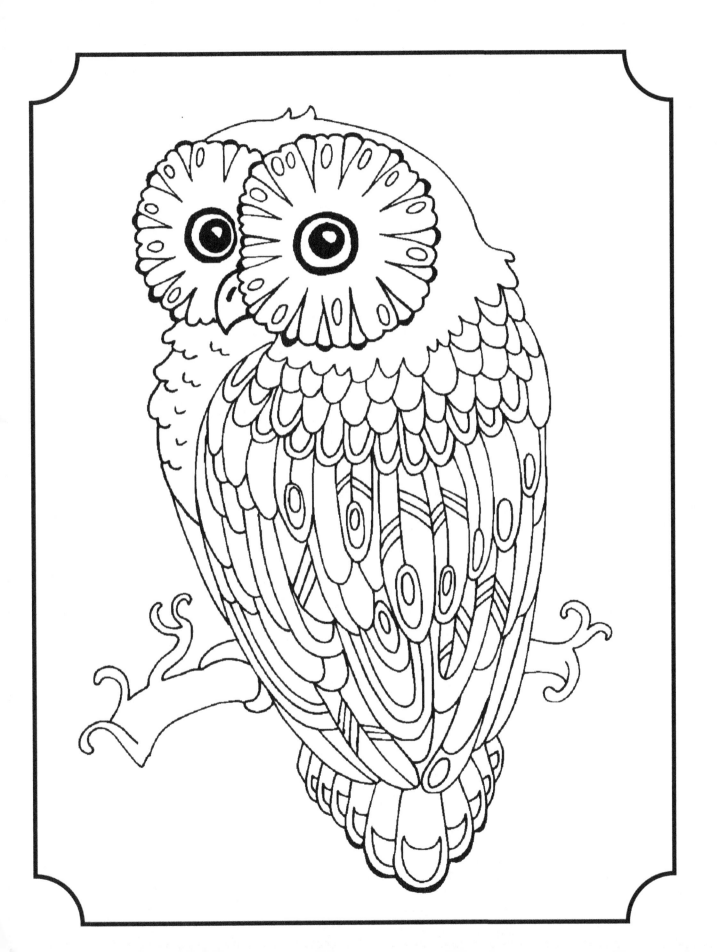

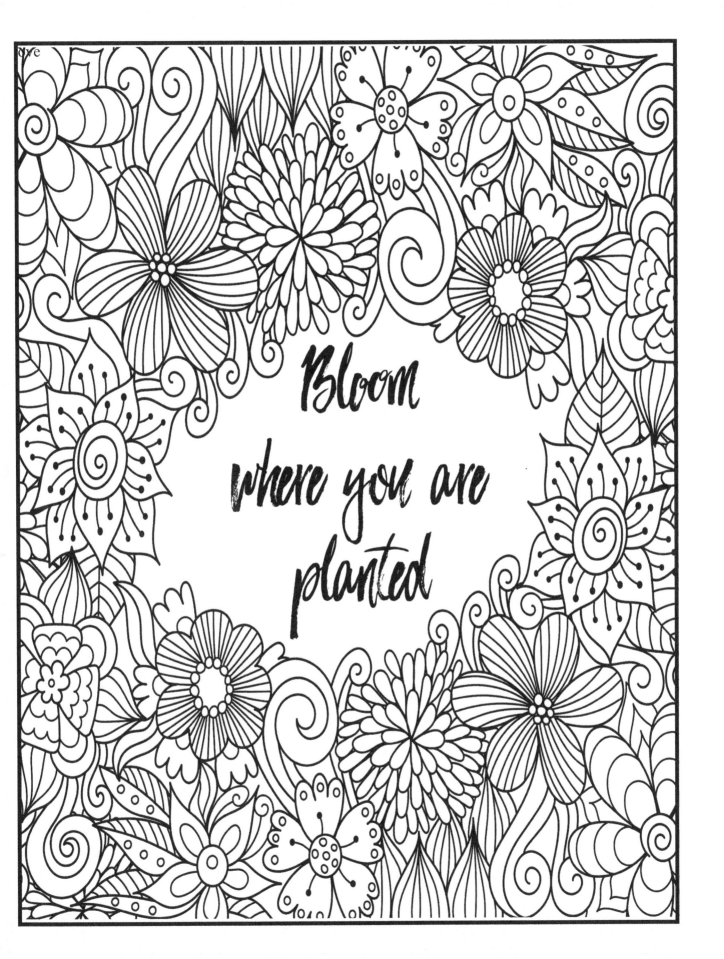

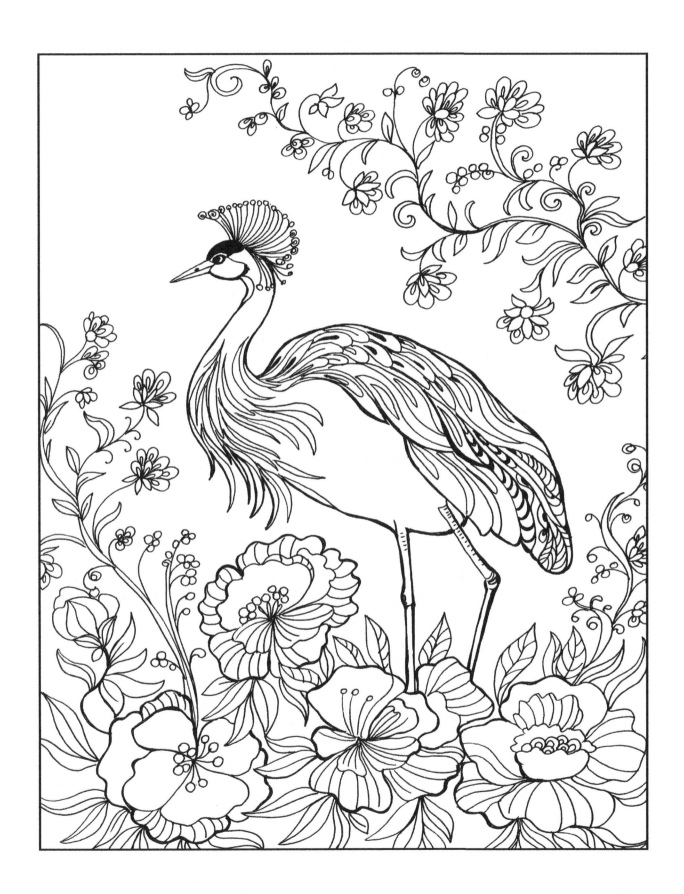

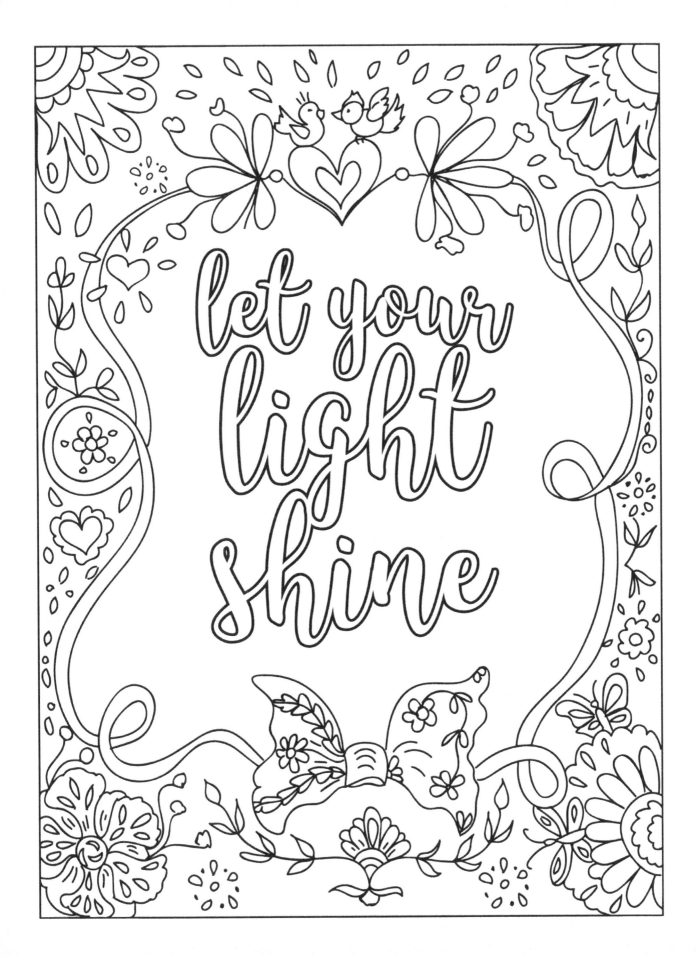

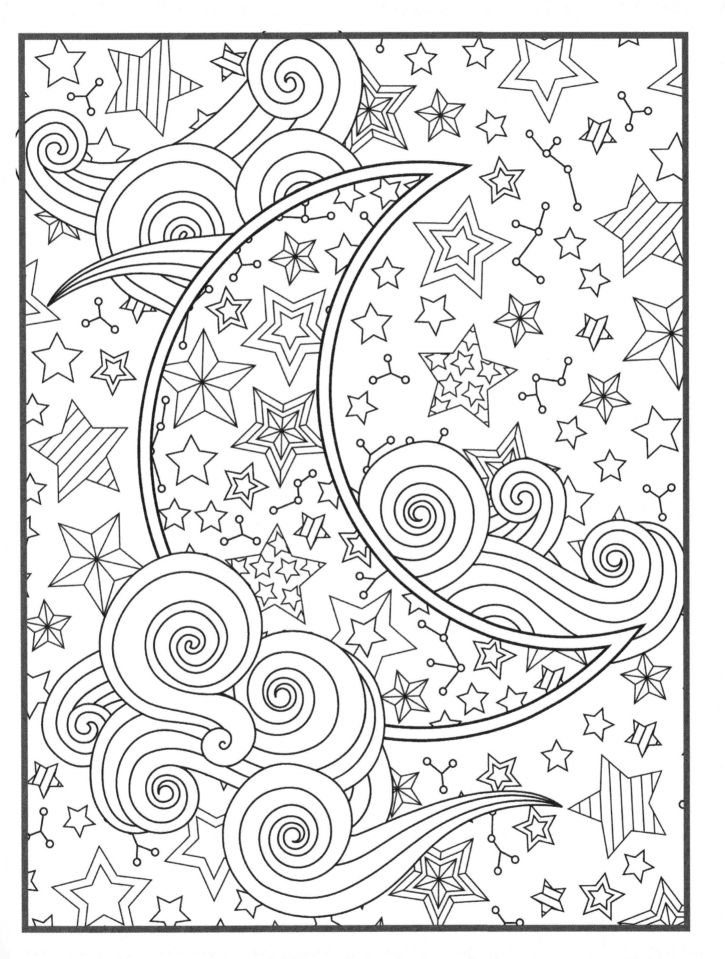

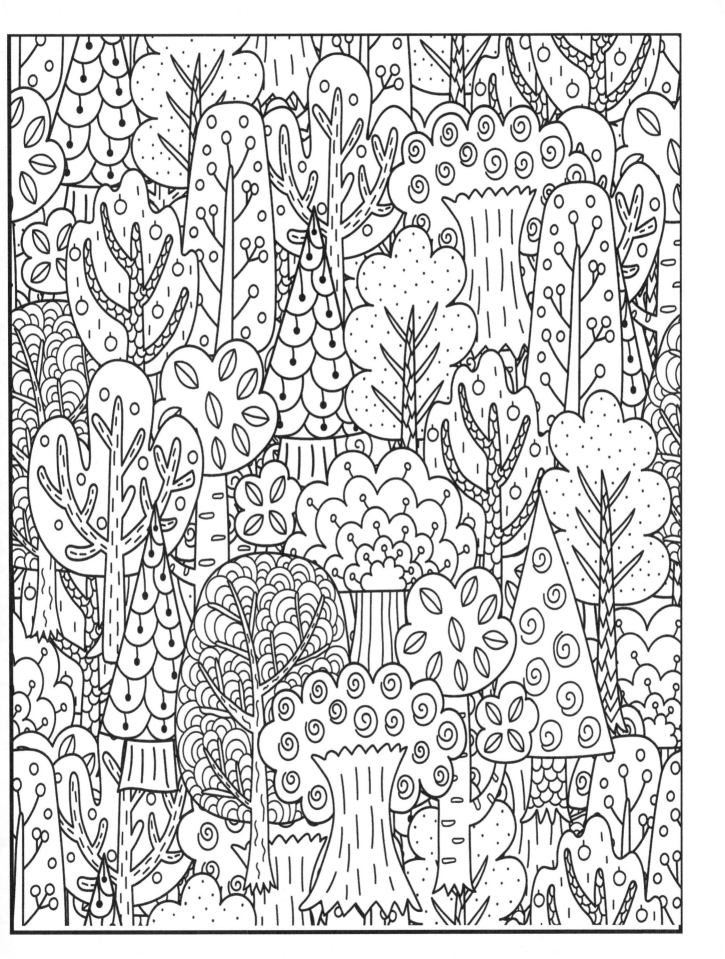

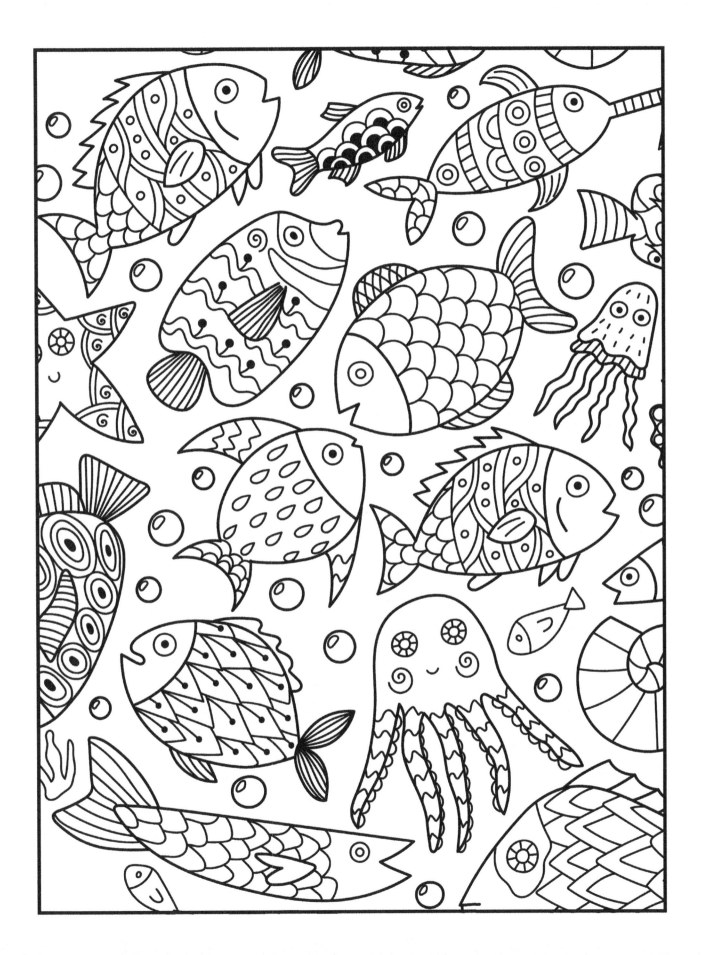

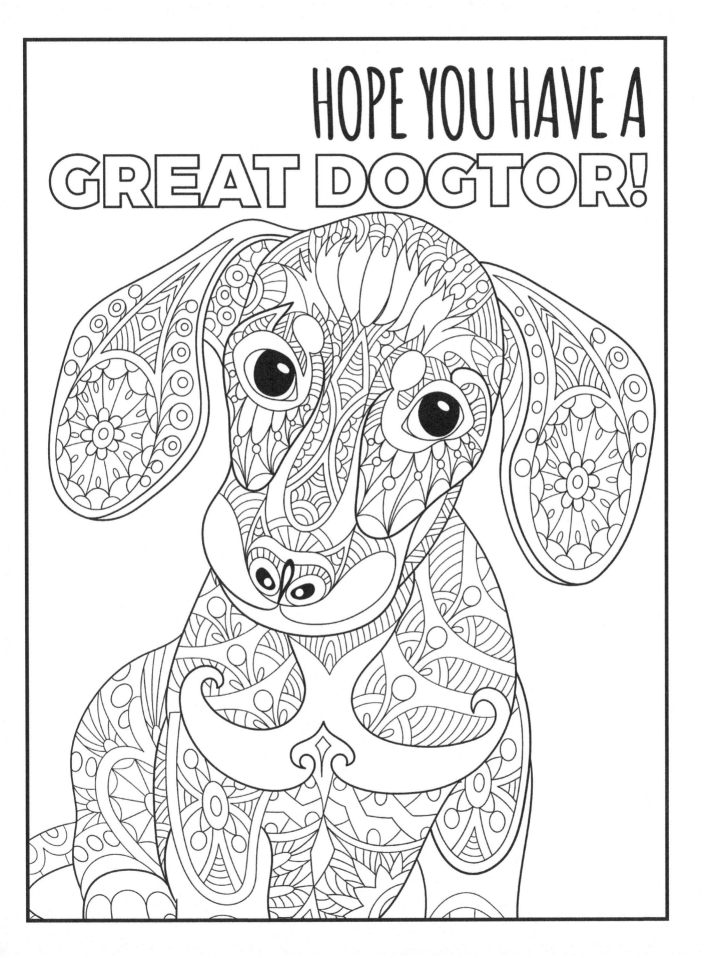

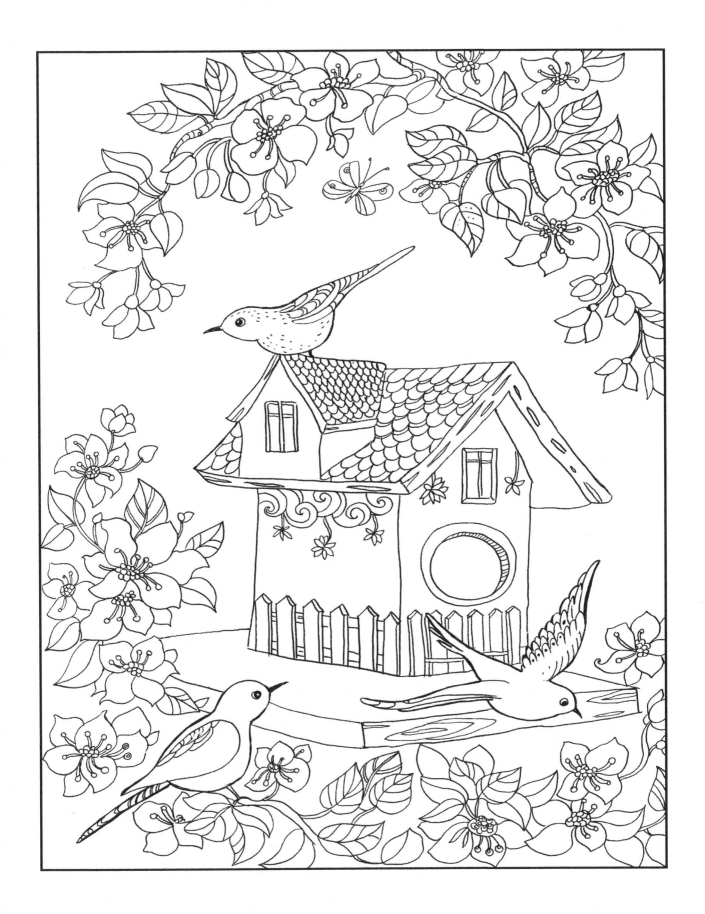

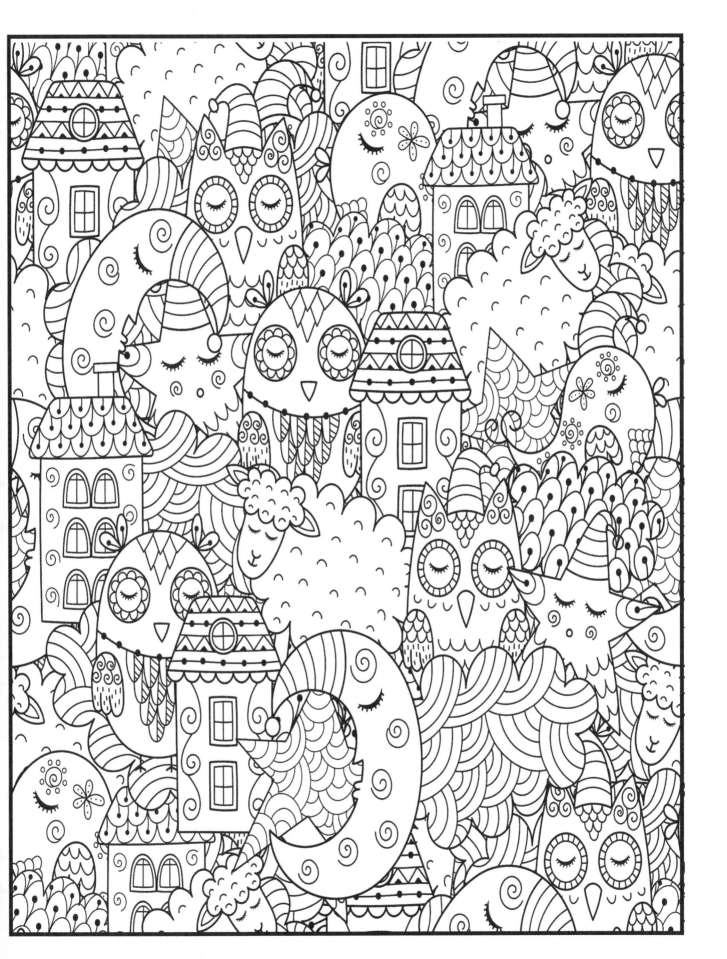

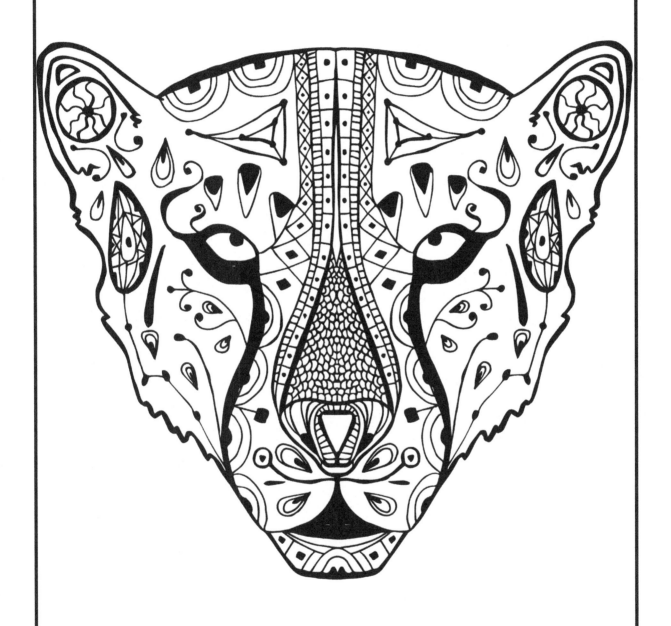

HOPE YOU HAVE A SPEEDY RECOVERY!

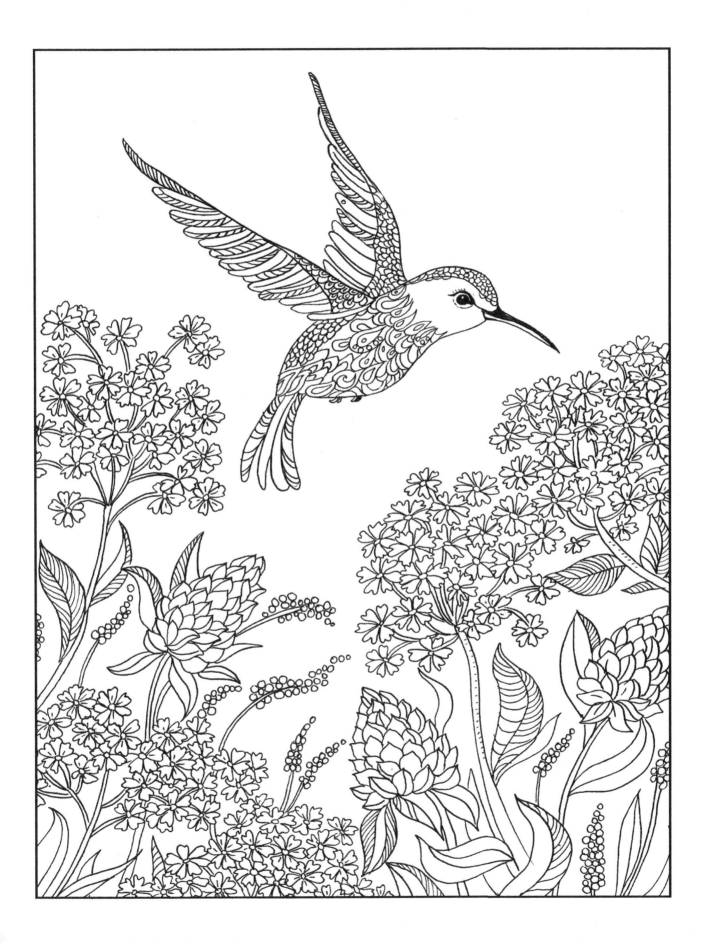

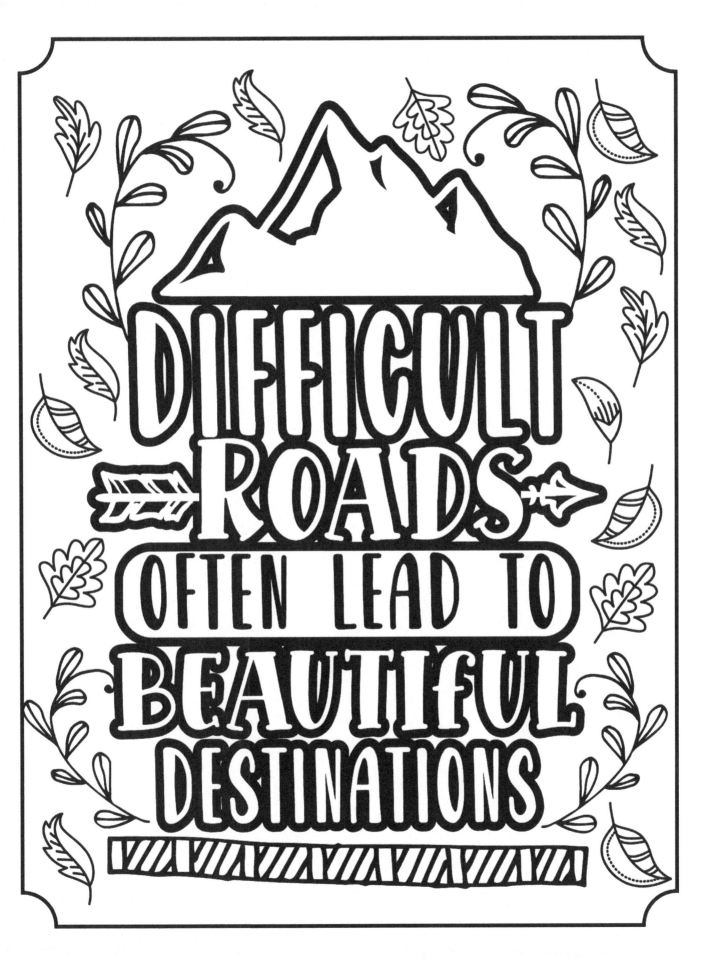

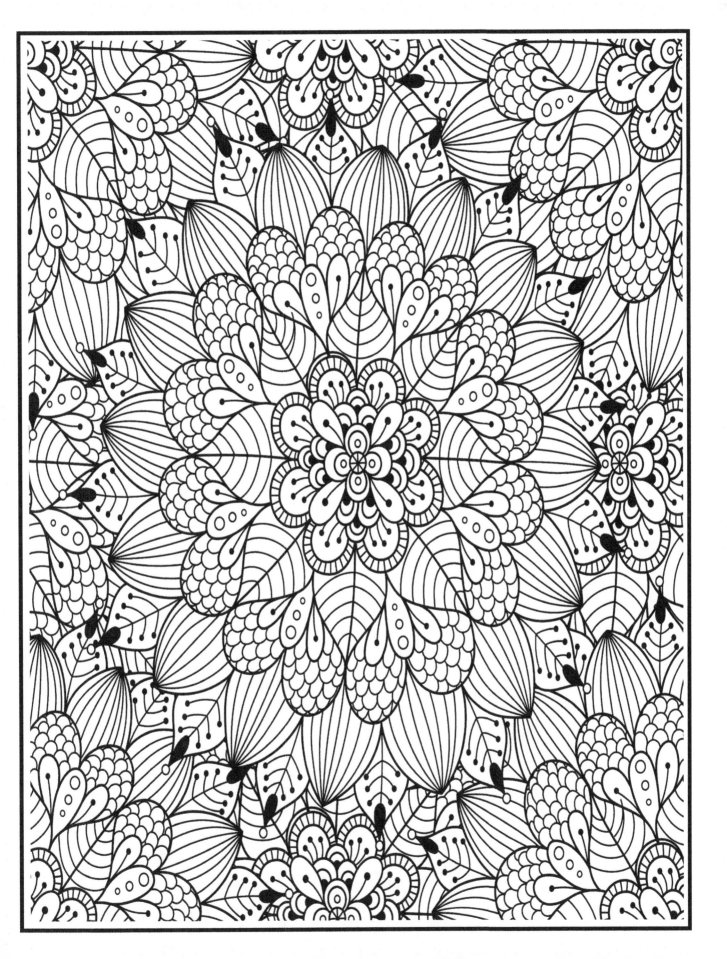

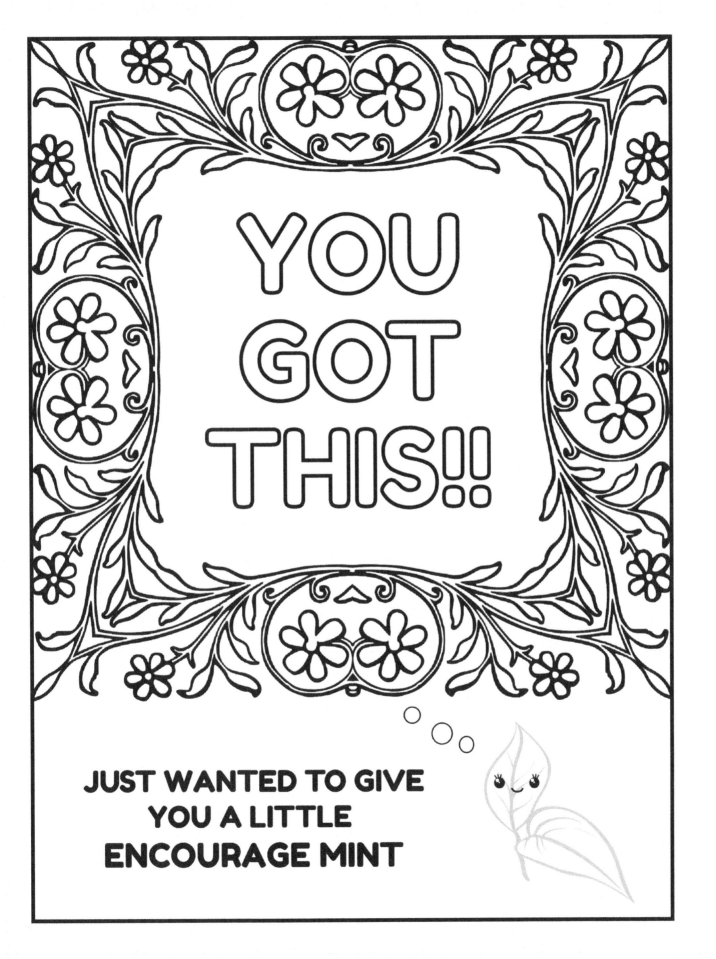

Made in the USA
Monee, IL
14 June 2023

35770173R10044